The Mini Neurology Series

Volume 4: Essential Tremor

Britt Talley Daniel MD

Copyright 2021 Britt Talley Daniel MD

Copyright Registered at the Library of Congress

Discover other titles by this Author.
Migraine editions 1 & 2
Transient Global Amnesia
The Mini Neurology Series:
Volume 1: Migraine
Volume 2: Carpal Tunnel Syndrome
Volume 3: Panic Disorder
Titanic: Answer From The Deep
The Mysteries of MacArthur Donne:
And If Thine Eye Offend Thee
The Case Of the Organic Chemist
The Spanish Flu 1918

With Amazon

Foreword

This book is dedicated to all afflicted persons and family members suffering from Essential Tremor. My intent in writing this book is to increase the understanding and knowledge of the treatment of Essential Tremor. Medical problems require human understanding, knowledge of which hopefully helps bear the suffering of the condition.

Britt Talley Daniel MD

Table of Contents

Chapter 1 History

Shakespeare Hamlet. Barnardo's line "How now, Horatio, you tremble and look pale."

In medical use the word "essential" means (of a disease) "with no known external stimulus or cause; idiopathic." Tremor comes from the Latin "tremere," 'to tremble'; "an involuntary quivering movement, a disorder that causes tremors and muscle rigidity."

Tremor is straight forward as to what the word means, but "essential" is a confusing term to persons not used to medical terminology. The word "essential" in medicine is used to refer to a medical problem that has no clear cause.

Thus, there is "essential hypertension" which affects 90% of persons who have high blood pressure yet the cause of the elevated pressure in this group has no known medical reason for occurrence. Earlier the condition was differentiated into "benign essential tremor" which came of no certain cause and "familial tremor" which had a genetic link in the family affecting half of children with tremor. Because the tremor causes symptoms and sometimes disability, the benign term was dropped and now the name is Essential Tremor.

The key features through time and discovery of the syndrome have always been a static, action tremor of hands, head, voice, trunk, or legs, which may or may not be inheritable, but little else is found wrong with the affected person. Neurologic exam is otherwise normal, and the condition was considered to be a monosymptomatic medical problem, but as time has passed Essential Tremor has been found to rarely be associated with dystonia, Parkinson's disease, Alzheimer's type dementia, gait ataxia, and deafness.

There are early references to tremor in Indian Hindu medicine called Ayurveda which exists from 4 to 6 thousand years ago. Both the Old and New Testament of the Bible have numerous references to tremor. There are also possible references to tremor in Egyptian medical documents from about 1200 B.C.

James Parkinson in 1817 first formally described essential tremor in his essay on the "shaking palsy," the illness that bears his name, Parkinson's Disease. He differentiated the differences between the two illnesses in his essay.

Louis, E.D., et al, writing about tremor in *Neurology* 71, September 9, 2008, pp 856-859 on "Historical underpinnings of the term *essential tremor* in the late 19th century," attribute the term *tremore semplice essenziale* (simple essential tremor) to Burresi (Italy 1874). Only a few years later, Maraglioano (Italy 1879), Nagy (Austria), and

Raymond (France 1982) described similar cases and proposed the terms *tremore essenziale congenito* (essential congenital tremor), *essentieller tremor* (essential tremor), and *tremblement essential hereditaire* (hereditary essential tremor) to define the illness.

Pierre Burresi was a Professor of Medicine at the University of Siena, Italy. He published a case conference of a man with tremor. Louis, E.D. et al, describes one of Burresi's patients:

> an 18-year-old man with severe, isolated
> action tremor. Tremor of the arms was
> present during voluntary movements. It was
> also present while walking yet disappeared
> during sleep. Head tremor was present.
> Neither parents nor siblings had tremor;
> hence, the tremor did not seem to be familial.

Louis, E.D., et al, end their article on the history of essential tremor with the following statement:

> "Beginning in the late 1800s. a number of
> clinicians began to provide a nosological
> separation for a tremor diathesis that was
> often familial and occurred in isolation of
> other neurologic signs. This disorder, which
> was named essential tremor, was later
> recognized as one of the most common
> neurologic disorders."

MacDonald Critchley (1900-1997), a British neurologist, described in Dr. Robert Joynt's obituary in the *Archives of Neurology* in 1998, 55 (1) as "an internationally known neurologist who was an enthralling lecturer and captivating writer. He was a bridge between the great British tradition of neurology, with representatives Walshe, Holmes, and Symonds, and the present."

Critchley wrote in *Brain*.1949;72:113-39, "Observations on essential (heredo-familial) tremor. His article opened with the following statement by Dana:

> "A fine tremor, constantly present in typical cases during waking hours, voluntarily controlled for a brief time, affecting nearly all the voluntary muscles, chronic, beginning in early life, not progressive, not shortening life, not accompanied with paralysis or any other disturbance of nervous function. Resembles to some extent the tremor of paralysis adjitans, still more a simple neurasthenic tremor. A most striking clinical feature is its hereditary or family type, and its transmission along with other nervous diseases." – C. L. Dana 1887.

> English neurologic literatures are almost silent about idiopathic or essential tremor (tremophilia, Zitterigkeit, tremor simplex) and its clinical variants, most contributions to our knowledge of the subject being in French or German languages. Merely from a perusal of the writings it is difficult to gain an idea as to the frequency with which essential tremor is

encountered. In its nature as a constitutional monosymptomatic peculiarity it can scarcely be regarded as a "disease," and some medical men might never have been confronted with an example. Some cases first come to light when the patient is called up for military service. For every instance coming to medical attention there may be a far greater number in which the victim does not seek professional advice. Moreover, of those cases where neurologic opinion is sought, only a portion are recorded in the literature. The milder examples therefore pass as a constitutional anomaly which causes little if any disability – a family trait perhaps. Other cases, where the symptom develops comparatively late, maybe incorrectly regarded as a manifestation of some clear-cut nervous disease, e.g., parkinsonism or disseminated sclerosis. When occurring in the aged, is often looked upon as an appanage of advanced years and dubbed "senile." – Critchley.

Chapter 2 Genetics/Epidemiology/Prevalence

Vittorio Alfieri. "Where there are laws, he who has not broken them need not tremble."

Genetics

Essential Tremor, also called ET, is an autosomal dominantly inherited condition which is progressive. Each affected individual inherits the ET gene from only one of his parents. Each child from such parents has a 50/50 chance of inheriting the ET gene. The abnormal gene can be inherited from either parent or can be the result of a new mutation in the affected person.

The ET gene has "very high penetrance" which means that persons who inherit the gene are likely to have clinically apparent tremor.

Essential tremor affected persons also inherit other commonly accompanying genetic conditions, such as dystonia, writer's cramp, ET with dystonia, and Parkinsonism. These families also show "anticipation" of the genetic trait, meaning that it comes earlier in life in affected persons.

So far, three gene loci (ETM1 on 3q13, ETM2 on 2p24.1 and a locus on 6p23) have been found in families with ET disorder. Also, a Ser9Gly variant in the dopamine D3 receptor gene on 3q13 has been suggested to be active.

Persons with ET who have no family history of tremor are said to be "sporadic." Since 50% of persons with ET are said to be familial with an autosomal dominant inheritance, the remainder 50% are "sporadic."

The problem with this sporadic group is how accurate this estimate is. Many movement disorder experts have examined the mothers and fathers of affected sons and daughters brought to clinic for possible tremor and have found mild essential tremor type involvement in many of these unreported parents.

Joseph Jankovic, MD Professor of Neurology, Director, Parkinson's Disease Center and Movement Disorders Clinic, Department of Neurology, Baylor College of Medicine, Houston, Texas stated in a lecture on Essential Tremor that "100% of family members have ET."

Some small tremor may affect almost everyone, and this mild tremor seems to worsen with age like essential tremor does. Mothers and fathers who bring their progeny with tremor to the doctor for an opinion may not be concerned enough about their own tremor to see a doctor for it. Then their own mild essential tremor will not be recorded in neurologic studies.

These findings tend to nullify some of the sporadic group, who are mildly affected with essential tremor, making an accurate number of ET effected victims intrinsically inaccurate to a small degree.

Prevalence

An estimate of the prevalence rate of any disease is related to how the disease is defined clinically and how the individual cases are detected. It is a well-known fact that many persons with certain medical conditions do not report to researchers who are studying those conditions and therefore, they are not detected.

Essential tremor is the most common movement disorder and affects about 10 million people in the U.S.A. ET is often misdiagnosed as Parkinson's disease, yet according to the Nationalist Institute of Neurologic Disorders and Stroke, twenty times as many people have ET, as have Parkinson's disease. Ten percent of persons with ET later develop Parkinson's disease.

Age at onset

ET is not confined to the elderly. Children and middle-aged people can also develop ET. In fact, newborns have been diagnosed with the condition.

Researchers estimate that 4-5% of people aged 40 to 60 have ET. The incidence rate for people age 60 and older is estimated at 6.3to 9%.

The Mayo Clinic reported a study of the prevalence rate of ET finding a rate of 306 patients/100,000 population or a rating of 0.3%. However, this study only included patients with symptoms diagnosed by a doctor, and it is probably an underestimate of affected cases.

One door-to-door survey for essential tremor was done in Copiah/County, Mississippi which included only persons 40 years old with tremor of the limbs, head, or voice. They reported a prevalence rate of 410patients/100,100 population.

However, 2 studies reported higher rates of population affected: for India, 1633 patients/100,004 and for Italy 405 patients/100,000, or 0.4% for all ages.

Studies reported varied differences, but likely in the United States, ET has higher than 400 patients/100,000 and a large number in the states go unreported.

ET can appear at any age, but it commonly comes on during adolescence or in middle age (between ages 40 and 50). With ageing the incidence and prevalence of ET increases steadily. For the Mayo Clinic group annual incidence of new medically diagnosed patients was 2.3/100,000 for the population under age 19 and 84.3/100,000 for the population over age 80.

Gender

Males and females are affected equally for limb tremor, but tremor of the head and voice is more common in females.

Race

Few studies of this have been done. However, the Copiah County study showed a non-statistically significantly higher prevalence of ET in whites than in blacks. A New York study showed ET prevalence in whites of 3.1% and in blacks of 1.8%.

Chapter 3 Pathophysiology

Pope Benedict XVI. "Mercy is what moves us toward God, while justice makes us tremble in his sight."

A principal ET researcher, Elan D. Louis, MD, MS, has stated about the pathophysiology of ET, "No one has ever demonstrated what the pathology is in essential tremor. No one has ever demonstrated cell death."

Currently the exact cause of ET is unknown although studies have suggested it may be a neurodegenerative disorder. Postmortem studies have found degenerative changes in cerebellar Purkinje cells. Lewy bodies have been found on postmortem in the locus ceruleus in 8-24% of patients with ET, especially in ET cases that go into Parkinson's Disease later in life.

Alcohol has a pronounced toxic effect on Purkinje cells, yet alcohol improves tremor in affected patients. Many persons with ET use alcohol for treatment.

Louis, et al wrote in *Neurology* V 69, August 2007, p.515-520 on "Blood harmane is correlated with cerebellar metabolism in essential tremor." Imaging studies have found that overall brain function is damaged in ET. Recent post-mortem studies have shown alterations in (leucine-rich repeat and Ig domain containing 1 (LINGO1) gene and GABA receptors in the cerebellum of people with essential tremor.

Harmane is thought to be a strong neurotoxin and is found in the human diet in various items. Laboratory animals exposed to harmane develop tremor clinically and pathologically have destruction of inferior olivary and cerebellar tissue.

Harmane is described by Louis, et al, as being "most tremorogenic" and may represent cerebellar cell death. Gut microbacteria also create harmane. Harmane blood concentrations are dependent on another genetic linked process—cytochrome p450 enzymes. Inheritance of cytochrome p450 enzymes may sync with harmane metabolism.

An 18% loss of Purkinje cells has been found in 75% of patients with ET and this cell lost is believed to be "tremorgenic" according to Louis, et al, above.

HAPT1 mutations have also been linked to ET, as well as to Parkinson's disease, multiple system atrophy, and progressive supranuclear palsy. ET cases that progress to Parkinson's disease are less likely to have had cerebellar problems.

Holly A. Shill MD of the Christopher Center for Parkinson's Research at Sun City, Az reported to *Neurology 4Today* August 7, 2007, p 39 that "Essential tremor is pathologically heterogeneous. ET has both cerebellar and Lewy body pathology present. She reported a study where

12 of 26 patients at autopsy had pathological changes in the locus ceruleus, 2 with Lewy bodies. In eight of the 12 depletion of pigmented cells was evident and seven showed tangles. Nine of the 26 patients had some cerebellar pathology, three with superior vermian atrophy, four with cortical sclerosis, and two with Bergmann cell proliferation.

In 2012, the National Toxicology Program reported an association between blood lead exposure at levels <10 μg/dl and essential tremor in adults,

Deuschl and Elble in *Movement Disorders* V 24, 2009, p 2033-2041 have proposed that ET is a cerebellar disease, due to abnormal oscillation in networks of nerve cells, "like a vibration in a car", that with time may damage the normal function of nerve networks that result in the symptoms of ET tremor and clumsiness.

Cerebellar degeneration has been proposed to occur with ET, a process not explained by clinical improvement of tremor with ET following the use of alcohol or DBS (deep brain stimulation) as treatment. PET scan of ET patients may show cerebellar disease.

It is possible that alleles of different genes will be found to be associated with ET clustering in different families and individuals. Understanding these genetic processes will hopefully lead to better understanding of ET and the development of new treatment strategies.

ET is its own distinct, yet idiopathic, disease or a group of diseases found together. It is true that some patients with ET develop Parkinson's disease, and some other neurological disorder. 23% of Dystonia patients have ET, and there is a modest association of ET with Alzheimer's type dementia. Most other patients with ET have no other similar comorbidities.

Conclusion: Most persons with ET have only the tremor although there is a rare association with Parkinson's disease, Alzheimer's disease, and dystonia. Neuropathologic exam of ET may show nigro-striatal degeneration, cerebellar atrophy, and Lewy bodies. The exact pathophysiology of ET is yet to be determined.

Chapter 4 Clinical Characteristics

Thomas Jefferson. "I tremble for my country when I reflect that God is just; that his justice cannot sleep forever."

General findings

Examining a patient with tremor means mainly differentiating between the two most common types of tremor—Essential Tremor (ET) and Parkinson's Disease (PD). The following neurologic exam comments are written from this perspective.

Hand tremor with ET is present during maintenance of a position (postural tremor) and during active movements (kinetic tremor). ET mainly presents with only action tremor while PD tremor is mostly a rest tremor. Parkinson's disease has motor symptoms consisting of a symptom triad of tremor, rigidity, and bradykinesia.

PD has non-motor symptoms that may come before the motor symptoms develop which includes sleep disorders, constipation, bladder problems, excessive saliva, dementia, depression, apathy, fear and anxiety, and cutaneous problems such as seborrheic dermatitis.

Benito-Leon A., et al, wrote in *Medicina Clinica* in May 2011 on "Neuropsychiatric disturbances in essential tremor" describing psychiatric manifestations in ET such as specific personality traits, anxiety, social phobia, and depressive symptoms which belittled the "benign mono-symptomatic" description of ET.

Type of tremor

The main clinical finding is that persons with ET have an action tremor, usually in their upper limbs distally, and rarely in their head, voice, or legs. The characteristics of an action tremor are that it comes with action on the part of the affected person; their hands shake when they perform some "action" such as writing cursive, shaving, drinking from a cup with a spoon, putting on make-up, eating with a fork, or trying to thread a needle.

The action tremor of essential tremor is involuntary and comes despite the wishes of the affected person. The tremor is worsened by stress and unconscious sympathetic adrenalin discharge. If Parkinson's disease is classically a tremor that occurs when the limb is at rest, essential tremor is a movement disorder that comes when limb is moving and performing an act.

Progression

In many cases, essential tremor affecting the hands or arms can slowly progress to affect other areas, most often the head. Although generally progressive, the rate of progression is slow on average. Recent studies have demonstrated that the average rate of progression of arm

tremor severity is approximately 1.5 to 5% per year.
Progression with ET mainly involves increase in amplitude.

The neurologic exam

Diagnosis of essential tremor or Parkinson's disease
is mainly through the neurologic exam; both require a
clinical diagnosis. The neurologist assesses the degree of
freedom of movement of the limbs of his patient, by first
watching the way he uses his hands, arms, and legs while
sitting comfortably and obtaining his patient's history.

During the neurologic exam he will watch his patient
walk freely away, turn around, and then return to him. The
patient will be directed to walk tandem, one foot in front of
the other, in an imaginary straight line, the policeman's
"drunk driver test."

The neurologist will observe the equality of the
patient's arm swings as he walks away, because Parkinson's
disease may start out with unilateral bradykinesia (one-sided
lack of movement) which later becomes generalized on right
and left. ET may be one-sided also, but not as prominent as
in Parkinson's disease.

The walking is often done in an office hall. Then the
neurologist may check for rapid movements of his patient's
fingers, hands, and arms by directing the patient to move his
index finger back and forth, from the doctor's finger to the
patient's own nose, with his eyes open or closed. He may

instruct the patient to hold their hands out in front of their body and to not move them.

Tremor

ET may join Parkinsonism in presenting with mild one-sided tremor. However, ET is classically an action tremor and Parkinson's disease a tremor observed at rest. PD typically is a tremor at rest but may also have kinetic and action tremor features. The unilateral tremor and degree of bradykinesia of Parkinson's disease becomes generalized with ageing.

The tempo of tremor with ET generally decreases with time, while the amplitude increases. PD patients may have a "pill rolling" tremor of rapid oscillation of the thumb moving across the base of the fingers. PD patients also may have a rotary, turning movement of the forearm and hand.

Then rapid movements of fingers can be observed by having the patient make tapping movements of finger/thumb, and one palm against the other palm, alternately with each side, right and left.

ET can also cause legs and trunk shake and some people have a feeling of internal tremor. Tremor patients may say, especially persons with ET since childhood, that they would hide their tremor by sitting on their hands or tucking them in their pockets to hide their shaking from the eyes of surrounding persons. ET patients like to avoid eating in public, and many times felt they were the only persons in the world who had such an unusual, embarrassing and disabling physical condition.

Remember that a slight tremor is found in everyone which worsens with aging.

Tone

Then tone will be assessed by instructing the patient to "relax" his muscles while the doctor flexes and extends his wrists, forearms at the elbow, and upper arms at the shoulder.

Tone should be normal for the ET patient in that there should be no rigidity. ET patients may have a perceived "cogwheel or rachet movement" to the limbs like that found in Parkinson's disease but there is no rigidity. Parkinsonian patients develop cogwheeling rigidity of their limbs, with resistance and a jerky rachet movement.

However, the patient's tone on analysis is usually completely normal for the "normal" ET patient; altered tone only appearing on the unfortunate patient afflicted both with essential tremor and Parkinson's disease.

Altered tone with rigidity and a "cogwheel" type halting of the wrist, or forearm movements is a marker for an extrapyramidal disorder such as Parkinson's disease. The Parkinson's patient has tremor at rest as his hands lie quietly at his side while sitting on the couch and cogwheeling rigidity of his limbs.

The essential tremor patient has tremor on back-and-forth movements of his hands and sometimes a cogwheel nature to the movements but no rigidity and normal tone in his limbs.

Free swinging movement of the patient's arms on straight ahead walking occurs normally for the ET patient, but the Parkinson's disease patient may present with obvious decreased arm swing on one side of his body, called bradykinesia. This reflects the reduced motor movement found with Parkinson's disease.

Handwriting

The doctor will have the patient sit and write his name on a piece of paper or construct an Archimedes spiral. The patient is instructed to draw a spiral without their hand touching a surface and the doctor examines the degree of tremor after this. ET patients have faster and larger tremor movements when they draw their spiral.

The handwriting of the ET patient is jerky and many times hard to read. The handwriting of PD patients is a small, cramped script called micrographia.

Symptom onset on one side

Both essential tremor and Parkinson's symptoms may be worse on one side of the body, later to progress to both sides of the body with the passage of time. The unilateral presentation of symptoms is more marked for Parkinson's disease. Many ET patients have noted their asymmetrical childhood tremor occurred on the same side that they developed Parkinson's disease rest tremor later in life.

The neurologist may grasp the patient's forehead on both sides and move the patient's head in flexion, extension, and lateral rotary movements, observing for rigidity, or cog-wheeling type resistance.

Dystonic posturing

The neurologist will observe for dystonic posturing of the hands with Parkinson's disease as the thumb may be unnaturally found in an opposing posture to the palm.

Gait

The young ET patient will likely have normal gait, turning and tandem walking. As the age of the ET patient advances, he may develop "gait ataxia," an often-unwanted accompaniment of essential tremor. The older patient may misstep on walking tandem and fall.

Parkinsonian patients develop a frozen, stiff appearing, bent over posture. They may have "gait freezing" at doorway entrances where they just seem to get stuck and cannot progress.

Posture

ET patients usually have normal posture, but Parkinson's disease patients develop a forward kyphosis with bending forward of the head, neck, and shoulders in a curved fashion.

Facial expression

Essential Tremor patients have normal facial expression for smiling, frowning, and general emotional response. Parkinson patients have a stare and "frozen facies" with a rigid, almost angry look, and decreased ability to express emotion as normal persons do with their smiles, grimaces, and sneers, that give ample expression of personality to most persons.

The Parkinsonian stare comes with reduced blinking and a bland, impassive, relatively immobile face. This frozenness reflects lack of motor movements of the muscles of the face, like the decreased arm swing on one side of the body in the Parkinsonian gait. It is referred to as facial bradykinesia or akinesia, meaning a lack of motor movement.

Development of Seborrheic Dermatitis in Parkinsonism

Many advanced, older Parkinson's disease patients develop seborrheic keratosis, which is thought to be a premotor feature of PD related to dysregulation of the autonomic nervous system.

Seborrheic dermatitis is a common chronic inflammatory skin disorder, affecting ~1%–3% of the general population. The dermatitis locates in sebum-rich areas, such as the scalp, face, hairline, eyebrow, glabella, nasolabial folds, ears, and upper chest.

The incidence of seborrheic dermatitis peaks for infants up to 3 months old, during puberty, and in adulthood. An incidence of 3.0% is found in men vs. 2.6% in women. Seborrheic Dermatitis is not a feature of Essential Tremor, and its clinical appearance suggests Parkinson's disease. The ET patient would have normal facial skin and lack the skin of the Parkinson's disease patient who may have seborrheic dermatitis with its shiny, greasy, acne appearance.

Longevity

There are long-held beliefs in the lay consciousness that Essential Tremor patients live longer than people without it. The Russian Neurologist Minor suggested in 1935 "that a factor for longevity was also contained in the tremor gamete."

A 1995 study found that parents of ET patients with tremor lived on the average 9.2 years longer than those parents who did not have tremor, leading to the conclusion that ET confers anti-aging influence and significantly increases longevity.

An explanation given for this suggests that ET patients have personality traits that encourage dietary, occupational, and physical habits promoting longevity. This needs to be studied further.

<u>Cognition</u>

Although there have been reports of senility or even dementia in ET patients, any cognitive changes ET patients may possess are nothing like the severe cognitive problems that come with Parkinson's and Alzheimer's diseases. Memory impairment in ET is only found after testing with sophisticated, sensitive tests.

The cognitive changes are "subclinical" and of little importance to the patient and their families. Also, ET patients, as mentioned are generally long-lived and old age normally has some memory changes.

<u>Hearing</u>

Ondo, W.G., et al, writing in *Neurology* on October 27, 2003 on "Hearing impairment in essential tremor" in which they studied, "hearing in patients with essential tremor (ET) vs patients with Parkinson disease (PD) and normal controls."

Their conclusion was that: "Patients with ET have increased hearing disability compared to patients with PD and normal controls, which correlates with tremor severity."

<u>ET association with Restless leg syndrome (RLS)</u>

Familial RLS has a strong association with ET. Ondo, W.G. and Deiian, L writing in *Comparative Study of*

Movement Disorders in 2006 Apr;21(4):515-8 on "Association between restless legs syndrome and essential tremor" found RLS in 33/100 ET patients, mainly those with familial RLS.

Ondo and Deiian stated: "Overall, we found a very high rate of undiagnosed RLS in patients presenting for tremor, but unlike other "secondary" forms of RLS, this finding was also associated with a high familial history of RLS, suggesting that they share some genetic similarities."

Stress

Essential tremor gets worse during stress and improves when tension relaxes, and emotions die down. This is due to the internal, autonomic nervous system relating to the events of life and secreting adrenalin during stress. The common phrase about this is, "I trembled with rage."

Once all this neurologic data has been collected in the neurologist's mind, then thoughts regarding diagnosis come to the surface.

Neuroimaging

Dopamine transporter (DAT) is a biomarker for dopaminergic nigrostriatal neurons that can be used with Single-photon emission tomography (SPECT) with cocaine derivative tracers binding to DAT as a measure of dopamine deficiency.

A large-multicenter European DAT-SPECT study of cases with Parkinson's disease, multiple system atrophy, progressive supranuclear palsy, and ET cases and controls correctly classified 97.5% of Parkinsonian cases and 100% of ET cases.

Now there is a reliable, yet expensive, laboratory means of accurately separating Parkinson's disease from essential tremor patients. This type of testing is commonly used by movement disorder neurologists.

<u>Conclusion</u>

To end this chapter, one must reflect that the individual with essential tremor would have a positive family history of tremor half of the time; and that the tremor would be mainly an action tremor which would progress slowly with ageing. The ET person would have an increased risk of depression, social phobia, anxiety, and hearing loss. His memory would be basically intact.

The ET individual would sometimes have rest tremor which would decrease when supine, and possible voice, head, and leg tremor in addition to the required action type arm tremor.

The ET patient would have normal posture, with no stare and normal facial movements, and intact blinking. Having ET may sometimes bring a cogwheel component to his arm movement but no rigidity. He would have normal tone in his limbs. He might have a slight tendency to fall due to ataxia.

He would not have seborrheic dermatitis, a diathesis, immediately marking the tremulous patient as having Parkinson's disease. The ET patient would also have a slight risk of developing Parkinson's disease as he grew older.

Chapter 5 Differential Diagnosis

Charles Bukowski "We are here to laugh at the odds and live our lives so well that Death will tremble to take us."

The usual differential Diagnosis is between Essential Tremor (ET) and Parkinson's Disease (PD), although there may be other diseases to consider. A full list of the conditions that should be in the clinician's mind while seeing a clinical case of tremor would be:

Essential Tremor

Parkinson's Disease

Alzheimer's Disease in older persons with essential tremor.

Multiple System Atrophy—a neurodegenerative disease with rigidity, tremor, dementia, trouble looking up.

Psychogenic Disease—previously called Neurotic, also called functional, meaning origin is from psychologic source.

Metabolic Disease-Hyperthyroidism—usually presents with goiter, called Graves' disease.

Cerebellar Diseases with intention tremor—a broad, low frequency, <5 Hz tremor which develops while visually guiding a hand to its target, hence intention tremor.

Dystonic Tremor

Alcohol abuse or withdrawal--delirium tremens.

Mercury poisoning

Liver or Kidney failure

Physiological Tremor—10 cycles per second tremor in normal persons stressed by anxiety or fatigue; common in rock-climbing where it is called "Elvis leg" or "sewing machine leg."

Wilson's Disease—disabling tremor in inherited metabolic disease-causing copper to increase in brain and liver.

Orthostatic Tremor—neurologic disease with tremor and ataxia while standing on legs.

Holmes Tremor--Rubral Tremor in Brainstem Lesions—upper arm wing-beating tremor, described by Gordon Holmes 1904, due to cerebellar stroke or lesion.

Neuropathic Tremor—an ET like tremor, more distal, postural, kinetic, and jerkier.

Multiple Sclerosis—arm tremor which may be mild or severe and disabling. "MS clumsy hand."

Stroke—especially stroke of cerebellum or midbrain fibers.

Traumatic Brain Injury—especially with damage to cerebellum.

<u>Panic Disorder</u>—tremor is a cardinal symptom of panic attack/disorder, due to adrenalin discharge. <u>Certain medicines</u>--asthma medication (sympathomimetic bronchodilators), amphetamines, caffeine, corticosteroids, and antidepressants and major tranquilizers used for psychiatric and neurological disorders.

Chapter 6 Types of Tremor

Lauren Bacall. I used to tremble from nerves so badly that the only way I could hold my head steady was to lower my chin practically to my chest and look up at Bogie. That was the beginning of The Look."

Rest Tremor. This is typically found in PD but cases with ET may have it as well. It has been called "pill rolling" tremor. It is a tremor which fulfills its name; the tremor comes with rest of a limb, in a limb undergoing no voluntary muscular activity. A rest tremor might be observed in someone sitting on a couch with their arms at their sides.

Action Tremor. This is a type of tremor that comes with movement and can be divided into: Postural, Kinetic, and Intention tremor.

Postural tremor comes when raising the arm or leg or the head still and quiet and against gravity.

Kinetic tremor occurs with voluntary motor movement, such as writing, eating.

Intention tremor occurs with goal-directed movement such as finger-nose-finger movement and the tremor intensity increases as the limb nears its goal.

Essential Tremor. This is typically an action type tremor with kinetic features. However, ET can coexist with PD and then would have mixed kinetic and rest features.

Parkinson's Disease tremor. PD typically is a tremor at rest but can also mix with ET and have kinetic and action tremor features.

Alzheimer's Disease tremor. ET may be commonly found with dementia and ageing, especially dementia in persons over 65 years old. An ancient medical term here was "Senile ET" where memory loss and prominent action tremor coexist.

Mixed PD and AD tremor. Some older, chronic, end stage demented Alzheimer's patients develop rigidity and bradykinesia which looks like Parkinson's Disease. PD and AD end stage patients may look alike.

Rate of tremor oscillation.

Oscillation here refers to the periodic count of the number of phases of tremor movement per incident of time. Tremors are usually defined in hertz (Hz) 1 cycle/second.

Quantitative analysis of these tremors can be detected in the electromyography lab with the use of electrodes placed on top of or inside muscles with a needle and then measured with an oscilloscope screen. These two tests are called accelerometry and surface electromyography.

Essential tremor usually has an oscillation rate of 4-12 Hz. Parkinson's disease has a rhythmic tremor rate of 4-6 Hz.

Chapter 7 Essential Tremor vs. Parkinson's Disease

Robert E. Lee. "I tremble for my country when I hear of confidence expressed in me. I know too well my weakness, that our only hope is in God."

Together ET and PD represent the two most common tremor disorders in adults. It can be a challenge to distinguish ET from PD, especially early in the disease when clinical signs may be subtle. It has been found that 1/3 of patients diagnosed as ET were misdiagnosed, with PD being the accurate diagnosis.

ET has been previously considered to be a monosymptomatic illness presenting with action tremor alone, yet 3% of patients diagnosed with ET later developed PD. In reported cases the time between onset of ET and later development of PD was 8 years.

There are two sets of criteria used for diagnosis of ET. The Movement Disorder Society requires the presence of persistent, bilateral postural tremor of the forearms. Kinetic tremor may be present but is not necessary for diagnosis. No other abnormal neurologic signs may be present except for Froment's maneuver, which is cogwheel phenomenon without rigidity.

Other criteria proposed by Washington Heights-Inwood Genetic Study of Essential Tremor requires the presence of moderate amplitude, postural tremor, as well as kinetic tremor, which results in impairment activities of daily living.

The UK Parkinson's Disease Society Brain Bank criteria require postmortem confirmation for the diagnosis of definite PD. The diagnosis of probable PD requires bradykinesia and one of the following additional features: rigidity, 4-6-hertz rest tremor, postural instability (not caused by primary visual, vestibular, cerebellar, or proprioceptive dysfunction).

The National Institute of Neurological Disorders and Stroke (NINDS) the criteria for PD only include clinical criteria for possible PD which require four of the following criteria: rest tremor, bradykinesia, rigidity, or asymmetric onset.

Yet, despite these well delineated criteria there are still grounds for confusion between Parkinson's disease and essential tremor. Patients with essential tremor may also present with Parkinson's disease findings, and vice versa. One of the confusing issues would be consideration of rest tremor.

<u>Rest tremor</u>

Rest tremor is a cardinal symptom of Parkinson's disease and if the patient also has bradykinesia and rigidity, Parkinson's disease would be high on the list of diagnoses.

Ninety percent of Parkinson's disease patients have rest tremor in clinical series and in postmortem studies of Parkinsonian patients it occurs in 76-100%. ET patients may have rest tremor in the arm, contrasting with PD patients where rest tremor occurs in the arm, leg, or both. These statements deal with the misperception that rest tremor equals or diagnoses PD.

Action tremor

Another perspective is that action tremor equals ET and not PD. Yet action tremor may also be found in patients with PD, some studies showing this is as high as 88-92%. Another misperception is that the tremor of ET is bilateral and asymmetric, but ET tremors are usually bilateral and mildly worse on one side, or else equal.

Head tremor

Since head tremor may be found in ET, there has been a question if it could occur in PD. The head tremor of ET occurs 4-6 times more likely in women than in men and is a postural tremor that goes away at rest, such as lying supine.

Head tremor also occurs in PD patients and will persist at rest, such as lying down. Head tremor was found in a community ET study 12%, 37% in a movement disorder referral practice, and 54% in a brain repository.

One study found head tremor in 17% of clinically diagnosed PD cases.

Jaw tremor

A rest type jaw tremor is typically found with PD, usually when the patient's mouth is closed, at rest. But jaw tremor can also be found in ET cases, 8% in a population sample, 10% in a tertiary referral sample, and 18% in a brain repository sample. For ET patients the jaw tremor was a postural tremor occurring during voluntary mouth opening or a kinetic tremor occurring while speaking.

Jaw tremor comes with older age, increased degree of arm tremor and with the presence of head and voice tremor.

Voice tremor

ET speech has a periodic or rhythmic modulation of either frequency (pitch) or intensity (loudness) in the voice. This ET tremor effect is noted especially during prolongation of a vowel. Voice halting or stoppage occurs with ET speech.

Sulicia and Louis, wrote on "Clinical Characteristics of Essential Voice Tremor: A Study of 34 Cases," in the *Laryngoscope* 120: March 2010, page 516-528. The authors stated:

> Essential voice tremor is a disorder of
> variable severity as it almost always involves
> a variety of muscles of the phonatory
> apparatus, both laryngeal and extra laryngeal.

It is most commonly seen in older individuals but may occasionally affect people in their second and third decade as well. Based on a group of patients seeking treatment, it appears to affect far more women than men and 1/3 to ½ of affected individuals have a family history of tremor.

About half of the cases occur with upper extremity tremor no more severe than that seen in similarly aged normal individuals, contrary to what has been thought to date. Essential voice tremor is probably more common than is generally suspected, and many cases appear to be undiagnosed many years after onset or are frankly misdiagnosed, most often as spasmodic dysphonia.

Patients complain of voice, instability, decreased intelligibility, and increased phonatory effort. The salient feature of essential voice tremor is kinetic (action-induced) tremor of the muscles of the larynx, pharynx, palate, and/or tongue and an absence of rigidity, bradykinesia, and spasms typical of other disorders of involuntary motion. The tremor produces rhythmic fluctuations in voice intensity and/or pitch and the extent and severity of the tremor relates directly to patients' local disability.

There is no evidence of efficacy of pharmacological treatment, including agents commonly used in other manifestations of essential tremor. Botulinum toxin is helpful to the majority of patients, but the benefit is typically incomplete and by no means universal, probably because of the factors related to the pathophysiology of essential tremor.

The voice of the PD patient is low volume and rapid. PD speech is said to be a hypokinetic dysarthria. It is monotonous and mumbling.

<u>Bradykinesia</u>

Bradykinesia is usually considered to be a cardinal sign of PD although some studies have found it with ET patients also.

Chapter 8 Pharmacologic and Neurosurgical Treatment

Jane Welsh Carlyle. "Does not a man physically tremble under the mere look of a wild beast or fellow-man is stronger than himself?"

Now there are multiple drugs for the treatment of essential tremor. There is no cure for essential tremor, but there are treatments that give relief and improve quality of life. These treatments include drug therapies and surgical procedures. The treatment chosen will depend on the severity of the tremor and the side effects of each treatment.

T A Zesiewicz, et al, writing on "Evidence-based guideline update: treatment of essential tremor: report of the Quality Standards subcommittee of the American Academy of Neurology," in *Neurology.* 2011 Nov 8;77(19):1752-5 has proposed the use of the following treatments:

Level A established as effective.

propranolol

primidone

Level B, probably effective.

alprazolam

atenolol

gabapentin

sotalol

topiramate

Level C, possibly effective

nadolol

nimodipine

clonazepam

botulinum toxin A

Medical Devices

MRI-guided ultrasound thalamotomy.

Gamma knife thalamotomy

This committee felt that levetiracetam and 3,4-diaminopyridine probably did not reduce limb tremor in ET and should not be considered.

Flunarizine possibly has no effect in treating limb tremor and ET and may not be considered. (level C) There is insufficient evidence to support or refute the use of pregabalin, Zonisamide, or clozapine as treatment for ET. (level U)

ET is the most common of all movement disorders and often affects the activities of daily living, including writing and eating. Propranolol and primidone are the medications used most frequently and successfully to treat ET. Propranolol is the only drug of all on the list that has been approved by the FDA for treatment of ET.

It has been found that 30% to 50% of persons will not respond to either propranolol or primidone and other drugs must be tried.

Comments regarding individual drugs

Level A Drugs. Propranolol and Primidone are the most common drugs used for treatment of ET, trying them first as monotherapy and then using both drugs together.

Propranolol is a beta-blocker medication first approved for preventive treatment of Migraine in 1974. Later it was approved as Level A treatment of ET. Propranolol is the "classic" betablocker for ET treatment, but other betablockers such as atenolol, sotalol, and nadolol may be used. In general, if propranolol does not work, then none of the other beta blockers will work.

TAB 10 mg, 20 mg, 40 mg, 60 mg, 80 mg

ER CAP 60 mg,80 mg, 120 mg, 160 mg.

Propranolol Dosing. 120 mg/day PO divided bid-tid

Start 40 mg PO bid, Max: 320 mg/day.

Long-acting propranolol can provide once a day treatment. Hand tremor responds the best to propranolol and head tremor the least. Propranolol gives improvement in tremor for 50-60% of ET patients.

Primidone is approved for treating epilepsy and ET. It can be a very sedating drug, especially with first dosing yet, sedation decreases with time of use. For discontinuation of Primidone the drug should be slowly tapered off.

TAB: 50 mg, 250 mg

Primidone dosing. 50-250 qhs

Start 12.5-25 mg PO qhs, increase by 12.5-25mg/day every week. Max:750 mg/day, divide doses >250 mg; taper dose gradually to D/C.

Note: Primidone has a high rate of discontinuation by patients due to its side effect of sedation.

Level B Drugs

Alprazolam is a benzodiazepine drugs indicated for anxiety and panic disorder. It is a schedule 4 Narcotic with possible addictive features.

TAB 0.25 mg, 0.5 mg, 1 mg, 2 mg

ER TAB 1 mg, 1 mg, 3 mg.

ODT 0.25 mg, 0.5 mg. 1 mg, 2 mg.

Start with 0.25 mg TAB prn tremor, may repeat in 4 hours. Go to 0.25 or 0.5 mg BID or TID for around-the-clock treatment.

Gabapentin is used for partial seizures, post-herpetic neuralgia, neuropathic pain, fibromyalgia, and alcohol dependence.

CAP :100 mg, 300 mg, 400 mg.

TAB: 600 mg, 800 mg.

Start with 100 mg or 300 mg TID, MAX: 3600 mg a day.

Topiramate is approved for partial seizures and migraine prevention.

ER CAP 25 mg, 50 mg, 100 mg, 150 mg, 200 mg.

Start with 25 mg/week and increase by 25 mg/week bid to 100 mg/day.

Trokendi XR and Qudexy XR

ER CAP 25 mg, 50 mg, 100 mg, 200 mg.

Start with 50 mg/day for 1 week and increase to 100-200 mg/day.

Alcohol

Alcohol has a prominent place in any consideration of treatment of ET because of its powerful effect on decreasing essential tremor. Many persons with ET have found that drinking a small amount of alcohol will temporarily cause a substantial reduction in their tremor. Some people have found that a single glass of wine or even one beer will reduce the tremor for 45 minutes to an hour.

In 1949, Dr. McDonald Critchley stated that for patients with essential tremor "a heavy dose of spirits will temporarily check the tremor." Patients with Parkinsonian or cerebellar tremor do not react to alcohol in this way. Following alcohol ingestion something like 75% of patients experience reduction of their tremor.

Thus, alcohol is the most effective drug for treatment of essential tremor. Propranolol and primidone, the most commonly used drugs for medical treatment of essential tremor, only reduce tremor in 50-60% of patients. Alcohol probably works through a central mechanism.

Use has been limited for fear of alcoholism. However, studies in Finland, Sweden, and the United States have found that the incidence of alcoholism in patients with essential tremor is no higher than the incidence in other patients with chronic neurologic disease.

Dr. William C. Koller performed a study utilizing a quantified approach with IV ethyl alcohol and found there was a strong effect of alcohol within the first 90 minutes after alcohol infusion followed by a severe rebound effect. Alcohol has a short-lived effect and exhibits rebound worsening of tremor after more than three hours and the next morning.

Alcohol responsiveness may be a key physiological feature of ET and understanding how alcohol works to subdue tremor may be helpful in choosing other drugs to treat essential tremor in the future.

Alcohol is helpful as a sorting out tool in differentiating ET from other types of tremor. Noting to a patient that if his tremor gets better with alcohol, he likely does not have Parkinson's disease or other neurologic causes of tremor.

It has been suggested that some patients could a enjoy glass of wine before dinner to reduce the tremor and make mealtime a more comfortable experience for them. Dr. Koller stated regarding the use alcohol for tremor that "it can be concluded that the occasional use of alcohol in ET patients is desirable and that the risk of alcoholism is quite low. Thus, judicious use of alcohol appears to be reasonable."

Botox treatment

Botox treatment delivered by a movement disorder expert provides statistically significant improvement in tremor. Successfully treated patients get injected every 3 months. Adverse reaction is mild finger weakness in about half of Botox patients. Botox works well for head tremor also.

Treatment for both ET and RLS

Control of both ET and RLS could be offered by clonazepam, topiramate, or gabapentin tried alone or in combination.

Medical Devices

Only patients who have had a considerable period of time of living with their tremor and who have tried an assortment of different preventive drugs should be considered for possible neurosurgical intervention. Most of these patients have been under the care of a neurologist or movement disorder expert.

There are potential side effects from neurosurgical treatment for Essential Tremor. A small lesion or area of destroyed neural tissue is made either remotely by Gamma

Knife, or, ultrasound, or by direct surgical lesion on an open brain. These side effects may be trouble talking, numbness in the face, and mild weakness on the side of the body opposite to the lesion. These symptoms are usually transient but may be permanent also.

MRI-guided ultrasound thalamotomy.

Deep brain stimulation is possible with a device called Neuravive. Neuravive is MR guided Focused Ultrasound (MRgFUS), a technique available to neurosurgeons utilizing focused ultrasound waves through the skull to target a specific brain area, the Vim of the thalamus.

This is brain treatment, without an incision or craniotomy. The thalamic Vim is the same target used years previously via an open craniotomy, which is a more invasive surgery. Tremor treatment by ultrasound and MRI localization can now be performed without an incision or anesthesia.

Gamma knife thalamotomy

The Gamma Knife technique utilizes MRI scanning for lesion localization and a focused beam of Gamma waves directed to the thalamus. This technique may now be performed safely for aging tremor patients who might have higher rates of surgical complication.

ET Patients are unfulfilled.

In spite of modern ET treatment as mentioned in this document many patients are still unfulfilled and have unanswered questions. Example of this was noted in the article by Lewis, ED, et al., in 2015 in the journal *"Tremor and other hyper kinetic movements"* 2015:5, where patients commented on what they are not getting.

In a survey of 1418 essential tremor patients, many felt that their issues were not being addressed:

1.1/3 of patients felt that their doctor was, not "moderately well educated" about ET.

2.lack of psychological service and support.

3.lack of physical or occupational therapy.

4.problem dealing with social effects of tremor.

5.feelings of not being in control.

6.lack of a detailed report in a more quantitative way of tracking tremor progression.

7.need of better counseling about current treatment and medications.

8.lack of empathy, compassion, and the feeling of being heard.

9 a treatment approach, other than just medication and surgery.

10.a discussion of all symptoms, aside from tremor such as cognition and balance.

Chapter 9 Useful information

St. Paul. Philippians 2:12: work out your salvation with fear and trembling.

The International Essential Tremor Foundation is located at PO Box 14005, Lenexa, KS 66285-4005 USA.

Tremor Talk.org is a blog on tremor.

Essential tremor.org is a website.

Facebook.com/international essential tremor foundation.

Twitter.com/essential tremor.

Comments from the book *I Can't Stop Shaking* by Sandy Kamen Wisniewski:

> Use an electric toothbrush.
> Tell the people at your bank that you have ET.
> Use credit and debit cards instead of writing checks. Use eating utensils that have large handles.
> Use a 1-inch-deep dish that has four sides.
> Hold your drinking glass in the palm of your non--dominant hand and steady it with your dominant hand.
> Eat with the utensil pointing toward you with as much twist to your wrist as you can manage.

> Comments from the International Essential Tremor Foundation:
> Essential tremor is a life-altering condition that

makes everyday living a test of ingenuity, perseverance, and self-esteem. Daily activities such as writing a letter, dressing, and eating cause frustration that can lead to stress and a temporary worsening of tremor. To assist people who have ET continuing to live full, meaningful lives this organization offers the following suggestions:

General

Learn to use your tremor-free hand for as many activities as possible, including writing.

Hold your chin towards your chest or turn your head to the side to control head tremor.

Use your tremor-free hand to steady your tremoring hand, and whenever possible, use two hands.

Avoid caffeine, ma huang, ephedra, and other over-the-counter medications and herbs containing ingredients that increase your heart rate and can increase tremor temporarily.

Keep your elbows close your body when performing tasks to help control him tremor.

Record notes on your cell phone.

Carry and use larger weighted pens and eating utensils.

Use a signature stamp when possible for signing your name.

Carry a strip of self-adhesive address labels to give to people who ask for your name and address.

Fill out deposit and withdrawal slips at home before going to the bank.

Consider using online banking to pay your monthly bills.

If you write checks, do them all on a "good" tremor day.

Consider using credit cards or debit cards instead of writing checks.

<u>Eating, drinking, food preparation</u>

When on the go, use lids for purchased beverages whenever possible.

Charry thick, sturdy straws with you.

Use heavier glasses and mugs instead of lightweight cups. Soup mugs are also a good choice for drinking.

When holding a mug or a small glass, place your thumb along the rim and place your fingers across the bottom.

Fill cups, mugs, and glasses half-full.

Request your meat be cut in the kitchen before being served.

Consider ordering finger foods to eliminate the need for utensils.

Ask that your soup be served in a mug.

Get a rubberized placemat that sticks to the table, so plates do not slide.

General practical tips from the July 2007 Neurology
Reviews written by Dr. Michael Sperber, a
psychiatric consultant at McLean Hospital in
Belmont, Massachusetts.

Tips for patients living with essential tremor.

Caffeine, amphetamines, and large amounts of
alcohol should be avoided. While small amounts of
alcohol may reduce tremor, large amounts may make
it worse.

Write using a heavy pen with a rubber grip.

Request to have food served in bite -sized pieces.

Use hook and loop fasteners instead of buttons.

Join a tremor support group.

Use an electric toothbrush and/or razor.

Attach light weights to wrists and ankles to provide
stability and decrease tremor.

Use weighted utensils when eating.

Use objects such as a table or chair or stabilizers to
help control tremor.

Use a brace during tasks such as writing or eating.

All the best.

Britt Talley Daniel MD

About the Author

Britt Talley Daniel MD is a practicing neurologist from Dallas, Texas. Trained in medicine at the University of Texas Medical Branch in Galveston and in Neurology at the Mayo Clinic, Dr. Daniel served his country as a staff neurologist LCDR, USNR at Balboa Hospital in San Diego, California at during the Vietnam conflict. After this he was on the senior staff as a neurologist at Scott and White Clinic in Temple, Texas, and an Associate Professor of Neurology at Texas A&M University Medical School. Moving to Dallas to start a private practice, Dr. Daniel taught at the University of Texas Southwestern Medical School as a Clinical Associate Professor of Neurology. Currently he is a member of the American Academy of Neurology. Married and with 5 grown children, Dr. Daniel is a lifelong folksinger and guitar picker. He is also the author of 6 medical textbooks: Migraine 1st and 2nd editions, Transient Global Amnesia, The Mini Neurology Series: Volume 1

Migraine, Volume 2 Carpal Tunnel Syndrome, Volume 3 Panic Disorder, and Volume 4 Essential Tremor. He has written a transgenerational novel about a medical family from England who relocates to America aboard the haunted Titanic, entitled: Titanic: Answer from the Deep. He has published 3 stories about a mystery solving physician entitled: The Mysteries of MacArthur Donne, Book 1 And If Thine Eye Offend Thee, Book 2 The Case of the Organic Chemist, and Book 3 The Spanish Flu 1918.

Please, if you read any of my books, review them on Amazon. I would really appreciate it. Literary Website: www.britttalleydanielmd.com

Twitter: http://twitter.com/btdaniel

Facebook: http://www.facebook.com/people/Britt-Talley-Daniel/1592670538

Migraine Blog: www.doctormigraine.com

Printed in Great Britain
by Amazon